Unofficial Guidebook for Preventing Cancer From Coming Back.
Or for: Living 3, 5, 7 Years More

Preventing Recurrence...

.How to prevent cancer recurrence for good cancers
.How to live 3, 5, 7 years longer for a bad situation
.How to avoid the same cancers for family members
.How to get old gracefully for family members or for yourself
- They are anti-aging lifestyles too
.Not to use supplements such as vitamins?
.Lifestyle interventions in this book are good for:
cancer-prevention for everybody
or just for good health
.Does low cholesterol causes cancer?
.These ways of life (lifestyle interventions) are showing: Powerful statisticsin the "Preface" on next page. One look at the next page:

I think you would agree they are effective like "<u>additional best cancer treatments</u>" But we still need standard treatments. They are absolutely necessary

"It seemed to amplify the chemotherapy effects many times for many of my patients." It's the author's opinion. And the patients' amazing cases are the proofs.

James C. Shum, M.D.
Medical Oncologist/Hematologist
Physician specialized in cancer care and blood diseases

Preface: Presenting the **Facts,** Raising the **Hopes**

Introduction: *Standard treatments have been improving over the past 40 years. There has been a 40% increase in cure-rate for all cancer patients. This brings the cure rate to 70% of all cancers. So chances are good for any new cancer patients to be cured.*

But there are things you can do to improve the odds of survival. They are discussed in this book. Some are easy to do, some not that easy. They have all been solidly proven.

Listed below as you can see: These ways to fight cancer can bring you more than 50% chance of not dying of cancer. And there is a 40% chance of preventing cancer from coming back. These percentages are in addition to the standard treatments.

Now is it worth your sacrifice to walk a few hours per week, and not to snack which is the #1 reason for weight gain? All those things and more will be discussed in this book.

Please compare the numbers to "new" treatment studies that follows(More examples are in the book):

* *"New treatments"*. Everyday, this was what I read from cancer journals presenting new treatment-study results: "A few more weeks or a few more months to live" for using this or that new treatments. Although at times new treatments could bring miracle cures. But they appeared only once in a blue moon. The followings are some lifestyle- intervention reports from major world health-studies. These may let you win a miracle cure "right away":

* Moderate amount of exercise bring you a 50% decreased chance of death from cancer.

* The act of stopping eating when feeling 80% full prevents 50% of cancers. And decrease the chance of cancer coming back to you by 50%.

* Keeping your weight down let you have 30 to 40% less cancer coming back (recurrence).

* Relax your mind and stress yields a 59% decrease in death risk from breast cancer.
* Checking your vitamin D level in the blood: Because it was estimated that 50,000 to 70,000 lives are lost to cancer per year when their vitamin D level was low in the US alone.

* Avoid sugar like table sugar: Sugar supplies the energy for all cells in our body. Cancer cells need a lot more energy for maintenance or growth. Lacking enough energy, they may re-cycle themselves by a program in every cell. The program is called apoptosis (recycling).

* Others: Hopefully more new molecular/genetic treatments would come. Quite a few so called terminal cancers have been made non-terminal with these new treatments. Or even complete cures have been achieved. (Topic will not be discussed in this book).

Did this information raise your hopes?
Doing them altogether, the effect should be at least as good as treatments, right? Or greater? Treatments improved by 1% per year. In one year, if you do the above lifestyle interventions. You are probably going to have 50% additional chance of beating cancer.

Table of Contents

Disclaimer

These "ways of lifestyle activities" or "life-style intervention-treatments" are as effective as treatments for treating cancer. They amplified the effects of chemotherapy many times. So they could be looked at as treatments themselves. But it is important and necessary to take your standard treatments which may include surgery, and/or radiation and/or chemotherapy. Together, they will be better in preventing cancers coming back for good cancers, and to greatly extend your life even with so called terminal stage cancers. The lifestyle interventions-treatments discussed in this book seems to multiple the chemotherapy effect many times. But its major role is helping the standard treatment, not instead of it. Please remember. These lifestyle intervention-Rx's would make you strong to take any treatments too.

But please note that just like standard treatments. The lifestyle intervention-treatments would not work a 100% of the time. But I pray sincerely these "treatments" would work for you.

Please consult your own doctor before you take up any of the recommendation in this book. Like some strenuous exercise is not for everyone. Or your vitamin/supplement level is already high enough that you really do not need them.

Any study results may be updated or even changed with time. And in rare cases, recommendations might change with time. Your doctor would know. Thanks.

Chapter 1
Introduction

Introduction: Nowadays, standard treatments for cancers are very effective. 70% of the patients are cured. But unfortunately 30% would still die. Why?

The cause of demise: The cause of death is due to the cancer spreading to critical organs like the liver, most of the time.

If the spreading is slowed down. The patient will survive longer. This has been a sure fate for most of my "terminal cancer" patients. Because the lifestyle intervention-Rx's discussed in this book <u>multiplied the effects of the cancer treatments many times</u>. It is here with these "intervention-treatments" that a "one-year-life" had been extended into 3, 5, 7 years for most of my patients. Making them like non-terminal cases. You agree?

There was not only one "terminal" stage patients lucky like this. The numbers were in the hundreds or more. Even 10 years survivals have been reported, orally from one doctor and in the internet from another doctor.

Prevent cancer spreading can prevent death. Hence if we prevent cancer from spreading. We would beat cancer and get the life back. This is the important thing for you when your cancer is so-called "cured".

Please assume that cancer could come back even when you are so called "cured". This cancer coming back could happen to some of the 70% so called "cured" people. It is a reality. Though fortunately, it would not happen for most of the 70% "cured" people. Especially now you have this book. You will see they can help you make sure your cancer does not come back (No recurrence). You probably will find out this is not an empty promise decades later.

Facts of life: You can beat cancer with these lifestyle interventions/treatments. Facts speak louder than theories. The fact is: Cancer prevention is a reality. You know hepatitis B vaccination have already prevented millions of people from fatal liver cancers. There are a few other vaccinations for other cancers. But for our readers, it is too late for vaccination-prevention talk. But it may not be too late to learn the wonderful power of lifestyle Rx's.

And preventing your cancer from recurrence is a reality too. Just see the facts now. Look at the facts section in each chapter. You can see how far the prevention of cancers from "coming back" (recurrence) is a reality. Its success rate is up to 40-60% with this lifestyle intervention-Rx's.

Read the case-histories about my patients. You can see real people enjoying the fight against cancer. You can see real people happily alive without cancer recurrence or be still alive years after years.

You can read about the patient who lost 3 pounds and had her carcinoid cancer disappeared from the left lung. It was from life-style "treatments" alone.

Or the chronic leukemia patient came out of the needed routine medical treatments, and yet controlled her leukemia change for years without restarting chemotherapy again. I retired. I wish it is forever for her. This is a first. Never seen this before.

Or two of my patients with myelodysplastic syndrome (MDS) who were supposed to die in a year or so, continue to survive and work for 4 and 5 years. They could still be around in this lovely world. I am sure of this even though I retired and moved back to NY.

The cases are limitless. Thinking back on their cases, my joy became limitless. This was rare in the life of a medical oncologist in the past decades. The older oncologists' souls had all been eroded by deaths after deaths of their patients. This is a different picture now. I am just happy I will not die a heart-broken retired medical oncologist when my time comes.

What to do to save your life: There are 6 main things to do. They all will strengthen your body against cancer. This one thing - "strengthening your body" would help you save your life. Or to greatly extend your life and time. When you can strengthen your body. You are not the same person anymore. With a stronger self, you may get rid of the cancer; or control it till the end..... When?

Instead of a year. The end may be 3, 5, 7 years as in most of my patients with "terminal" cancers. Or it could be 10 years as other doctors reported.

There is one most important item among the life-style items. If we do this item alone, it will make the body a lot stronger. It is to control your weight. To control your weight means you have to do a little exercise, stop eating when feeling 80 % full, and to avoid sugar.

Now you may just be reading through these words, not feeling excited that they can save your life. Wait until you read the chapters. You will be surprised with the facts and the cases. You will probably be a believer that if you do these things, you will beat cancer. When years or decades passed, and your find yourself still alive. Finally you will be a true-believer.

How true is the living 3, 5, and 7 more years? A primary care doctor told me," Dr Shum, your patients always come back." This certainly meant my terminal-stage patients were living well beyond their one year limit. They kept on coming back to their primary care doctors for medical follow-ups. There were so many of them, coming back years after years. The busy primary care doctors finally noticed that there was something odd. How could they live that long! Of course, they had no time to research the reason why. But they noticed.

This has been the best statement I ever got. Yes, the statement reflects the fact that my end-stage patients are really living years longer. What could have been better? Nothing!

I just wish they never die. Let me wish it upon you now.

So now, I hope you could put your worries away, and could relax your mind. Does relaxing your mind reduce the chance of cancer spreading? Little things like that?

Yes, it does, proven in studies. All these little things that can dwarf the devil called cancer have been proven by million-dollar studies. I beg your pardon. Quite a few of the studies have already cost more than 100 million dollars. Believe in them please.

No academic proof, however, is better than one cancer patient being alive, without cancer. Or the cancer seems forever controlled. And there are thousands of them --- totally cured, or alive at 3, 5, 7 years beyond their time. You could be one of them.

Thanks are to all those lifestyle interventions/treatments. And thanks are to all the researchers that brought these life-saving facts to life. And above all, thanks are to all the patients who believed, and practiced those "treatments", and benefited from it. Because they are doing so well, I felt I have done my job for humanity. And I am no longer depressed.

Now 1, 2, 3! Get up and do it. Learn them; do them, to save your life or time.

Chapter 2
Stress, Depression and Cancer

Introduction: Depression, a natural response.
It was just a natural thing waiting to happen. When we were diagnosed with cancer, we became deeply depressed.

My experience: In the year 2002, I had a small swelling in the bone in my left upper jaw. It was as big as a small chestnut. I became depressed immediately. For as a physician specialized in cancer care, I knew sarcoma at this location is deadly. It was promptly biopsied. You can bet on that.

Before the pathology report was available, I became a "dead man walking". My life left me. I was in shock. Like I said, cancer in this location is deadly. I could swear, nothing in this world could lift me out of the depression. After all, death was knocking at the door.

I continued to see patients with cancers, doing my best for them.

Things became different after the result of the biopsy was delivered. It turned out to be a mild sarcoma - a "desmoid tumor". I had a 90% chance of cure like other patients with good cancers. I instantly felt like I came back to the living world. The whole event made up a big chapter in one of my books:" *Who Isn't Afraid of Cancer*." in Amazon.com, under my name.

I had no worry right there, right then.

I knew I was going to live with that mild cancer. Other patients with cancers would not be as lucky. Because even with so called good cancers, they would still be worried. For they do not know how good or how bad they are going to be. This is a great source of distress.

To help patients in this situation, I wanted to provide a little pointer about how one is going to fair after the diagnosis of cancer. I designed a scenarios system for each cancer. Each cancer was classified into different scenarios. So if you look at the scenarios in the chapter of the cancer you have. You may then have an idea of how well you are going to be. It is also in the same 300 some pages book mentioned on page 15. I hope you would find it helpful. The book is in Kindle also.

I wish to make this current book slim, so it could be inexpensive. Please excuse me for not repeating.

How did my terminal stage patients do? When they knew they were going to die. Did they appear very depressed and looked like "dead men walking" like I was? Yes, they did. They walked in like people who were already dead. But that feeling only happened before seeing me the first time. Starting the second follow-up visit, they walked like normal people. Their eyes were full of hope. They all showed great resolve to fight their cancers.

What happened? It was simple. In the first consultation visit, I gave each patient a single piece of paper. It summarized what they could do to fight cancer. Those were the summaries of the "facts" in this book. They knew those studies were truly helpful. They believed the wonderful results of preventing cancer recurrence for people with good cancers. For patients with the terminal stages of cancers, they learned those methods would win them some time.

But little did we know most of them would win years and years of life back. Survivals were long instead of what was the usual - about a few months to a year to live.

My end-stage patients lived normal lives. Knowing they had a chance, knowing how to fight the cancer, their stress and anxiety were greatly relieved. They all looked like normal people. Now they had a direction and a determination in life - to fight cancer.

They did all the cancer fighting "lifestyle intervention-treatments". All the time, they were concerned with "weight control", "exercise", "stop eating when 80% full", "eating the right diet", and "practice meditation". And their minds were not obsessed with the fears of cancer anymore. Their minds were busy reminding themselves of doing the interventions to stay alive.

And in some of their minds was," If I gain weight, Dr Shum is going to talk to me for a long time". That perhaps was a greater fear than cancer. Believe it or not.

Anyway, doing all that had to be a full-time job. They had no time for sadness. They knew they have done their best. They have no other regrets. They left no time to feel depressed. Me and them as a team, we were having battles with cancers and we felt invincible.

We never look back. More than half of them with advanced stages lived years longer. When there is hope and there are ways to fight cancer, on top of the standard treatments. You see, there is little time for depression.

The best anti-depressant: So believing in the discussions in this book and doing it could be one of the best anti-depressants. As you can see in the above paragraph. Even in the face of having terminal cancers, my patients lived like normal people. We had a common purpose - to fight cancer.

And in the real world, academically speaking, "Exercise is the most robust ((huge) and long lasting anti-depressant known to psychological science". In plain language, that means exercise is the best anti-depressant. It lasts long. And the academics know it.

We will see cases and facts about exercise in the next chapter. Let's now see two cases of how depression could "cause" cancers in case #1. And in case #2, there is the case-history of one of my patients that I would not soon forget. I doubt I will ever forget.

Case-histories:

Case #1: This is a case of people with depression having increased chance of cancers.

This is a study of 5000 rather elderly folks. One group had depressed symptoms. The other group did not. Only a short four years later, the depressed group had 88% more cancer deaths. I think this statistics speaks for itself.

Case #2: This is a case-history of one of my patients. Having depression in this patient let a good cancer eat her right shoulder bare, showing bones. But do not lose hope. Depression can be lifted. And cancer can go away.

This was the case of an elderly lady. She had skin cancer. The skin cancer was just "basal cell carcinoma". It is generally curable and slow-growing.

But yet her skin cancer eroded her shoulder. So I knew at once there must have been a reason. It turned out, it just happened she fell out with her sister. Her sister was the only living human being she knew at her age. So she was very depressed and let the cancer progressed.

So I urged her to make up with her sister. And I arranged for the best treatment there was for her. She received combined chemo-radiation therapy at the same time. She was followed with the wound-care team as well. And she started talking to her sister on the phone.

Three months later, she came for follow-up. She had her normal shoulder back. And CT showed there was no cancer anywhere else. And she had been in good terms with her sister.

I learned from this case. Depression can turn a good cancer into a bad cancer.

A little advice regarding depression: Remember. If you want to win your life and time back from cancer. Your depression has to go. So now please look depression in the eye, and beat it. With all the suggested proven methods to fight cancer discussed in this book, you can easily make yourself feel <u>you are in control, not the cancer</u>. Even my "end-stage" patients lived like normal people, as we discussed above. So will you, right? Please read the "facts section" that follows. See how good "group meetings" can be and how mind-body exercises can reverse depression. Thanks.

Scientific Facts on depression and treatments:

* During chronic stress/depression, it is found out there are so called **stressed hormones** that remain at high level in the blood. These are the epinephrine and nor-epinephrine. **They were proven to cause cancer in the laboratory.** They help cancers spread too.

Mind-body exercises like **meditation were shown to lower the stress hormones down to normal. So the cancer-inducing environment can be reversed.**

There are lots of books in the library teaching meditation techniques. I learned it in one single reading during high school years in the 1960's. I described it in detail in my book, *"Run...Run Away From Cancer"*. Sorry I have to refer to other books. So this book can be brief and can be sold inexpensive. So more people can read this book and be helped from the damage that cancer brings.

*In women with the bad breast cancers labeled as "triple negative", beta-blocker which is an anti-hypertensive medication can also block the epinephrine/nor-epinephrine actions. The women on this medication had better survivals. Study is ongoing.

* Some news from a "Human gold-standard" study showing stress reduction influenced the survival times of breast cancer patients. This was a study of 227 women with breast cancers. Half of the patients were in the stress-reduction group, the other half just underwent regular treatments. At the conclusion of the study, the results showed stress reduction helped the survival and recurrence of the breast cancer patients.

There was a 45% reduction in breast cancer recurrence (coming back).

There was a 59% reduction in the risk of death in the stress reduced group.

Yes, like you, I exclaimed, "Unbelievable!". Just a little stress reduction can give us a 60% less chance of death. Please believe it. Please take care of yourself, and find ways to reduce the stress.

* In animal studies, the stress animals die twice as often - similar to the above human study.

* Stressed elderly people have weaker immunological response. This simply means they have a weaker immune system. A weaker immune system allows for more cancer to appear.

* Some evidence showed patients who are depressed do not do as well with treatments.

* In animal studies, stressed animals have breast cancers spreading to the lungs 30 times more often. The next three fact items are findings in animal studies also.

* Stress/depression: There are more new blood vessels formed by the cancers, to get nutrition.

* Stress/depression: There is more cancer spreading (metastasis).
* Stress/depression: The recycle program (apoptosis, or programmed cell death) is inhibited when stressed. So cancer cells don't go away by recycling.
* Even in patients with bad cancers, stress/depression can make survival difference too: This was a study of patients with bad liver cancers. With this liver cancer, patients sadly could survive in terms of only months. Yet the difference still showed.

In the group with depressive symptoms, the average survival was 5 months. While the group without depression lived 11 months, a whole half year longer when not depressed.

*Support groups makes a difference: Patients attended meetings in the support groups were found to have less depression. You know depression can turn a good cancer into a bad cancer. So if you lift your depression, cancer will be less bad. Right?

The American Cancer Society may have a website for support groups near you. The social workers or some old patients know where to find them.

A few words about cancer support group meetings: Most cancer centers have support group meetings. New patient can learn about treatment side effects and how to avoid them in the real world. Having someone in the "same boat" to talk to is very anxiety releasing. I will always remember an elderly woman supporting a young lady. She held her hands while the young lady was receiving her very tough regime of chemotherapy. The young lady thus was able to complete the whole treatment course and gained more than 3 years to live. How I wished it could be longer. Both were my patients. You talk about support groups. This is what it can do.

In the support group my patients attended, they exchanged their cancer-fighting experience in addition. Invariably, they learned about my enthusiasm to help them fight the cancers as a team. Those meetings usually made them more determined to fight cancers.

On the little fearful side, they learned that if they gained weight, they will hear a long talk from me automatically. I was very proud. Out of a couple of thousands of my patients, only one gained a few pounds. He was an elderly patient with prostate cancer. Some very elderly patients sometimes looked at me as if they were saying," What more do you think I want, Doc?" I sometimes scratched my head in helplessness with them. And changed the topic of the talk.

Main means to relieve stress and depression: These were the points we have discussed before. Now I just want to emphasize them.

1. Anti-depression medication is very effective. It reverses the cancer causing stress hormones proven in studies. Now these anti-depression medications can easily be obtained from the primary care doctors. Of course, psychiatric care itself could greatly help too.

2. Meditation among the mind-body exercises has proven to reverse the cancer causing stress hormones too.

3. Exercise is the best anti-depression medication. This has been recognized in psychological and psychiatric studies. I bet we know it without those studies. Please exercise.

My gratefulness for the lifestyle "intervention-treatments":
I was grateful that most of the patients were doing a whole lot better. That is the point of my gratefulness. This only happens when patients can receive the improved standard therapy plus the lifestyle "treatments". Their cure rate is not the standard 70%. It is much higher.

This has changed the dark and gloomy days of oncology of yesteryears, into the bright and sunny days of nowadays for me.

This has been so different for me now compared to the 1970's. In those dark days, the shadow of death of the patients dominated my life. What else could it be when 70% of your patients died in those old days. Gratefully, cancer treatment slowly, but surely improved, punctuated by near miracle cures once in a blue moon. But it still was not enough to lift my spirit.

The change for the better started with the news report of an old lady in China. She had terminal stage lung cancer. She failed the standard treatments, and was told to have only 7 months to live. She started running and finally successfully ran the cancer away. It opened my eyes to this running as another treatment for cancer. Though I was somewhat skeptical at first.

Later, my eyes were really wide-open when I dug a lot of information up from literatures. There are many lifestyle activities that are potentially additive to treatments for cancers. The statistics were unbelievable. *50% less cancer patients died. 40% cancer prevention.* Do you know what I got used to read from our new cancer treatment-studies everyday? "A few more weeks or a few more months to live". So you can imagine the results of the lifestyle intervention-Rx's must have blown my mind away like atomic bombs.

I have been calling these lifestyle intervention-Rx's. They were all from good studies. I hurriedly summarized them in a piece of paper, and handed it to all my patients. Since the chance of harm is negligible, but the potential benefit is so huge. I preached and swore by the studies and earnestly wanted them to try the lifestyle intervention-Rx's to beat cancer.

The patients believed in them and practiced them.

But both patients and I did not really know how strong all these additional "treatments" would be. Yes the statistics were great. But we just had to wait and see how it worked.

A few years later, my patients with good cancers never seemed to recur. The patients with terminal cancers were surprisingly still alive. They did not die at the one year mark! Most of them continued to live year after years! Oh my God, those lifestyle intervention-Rx's, on top of the standard treatments, did work. Those lifestyle "treatments" are powerful! Their much prolonged survivals surprised the busy primary care doctors too. They noticed.

These wonderful results in my patients were absolutely out of my expectations. Right there I knew these lifestyle "intervention-treatments" were powerful. I realized without doubt. They saved most of my patients. They lifted my spirits up.

Finally, I could come out of the dark gray world of oncology of yesteryears. My final years in oncology were bright and sunny. We had largely conquered cancer! The patients and I. Though there was still a lot more that needed to be done.

There are no words for me to express my thanks to the patients and the life-saving "intervention-Rx's". The patients' triumph became my joy. The cancer treatment world is a lot brighter when patients practiced these lifestyle "treatments". The cure rate is not the unsatisfactory 70% anymore!

There are no words really. There are no words that can express my gratitude.

Of course, I would be more grateful if you pick up these lifestyle methods (treatments) to fight cancers and benefit from them.

So for you, I have a question. After reading this chapter, do you want to take care of your depression or not? Please give it a try.

Chapter 3
Exercise, a Little is Ok, the More the Better

Introduction: Besides being the best way to get rid of depression, exercise also kills cancer too. We shall see how it could kill cancer in this chapter. Let me begin with a news report showing the power of exercise killing cancer.

A shocking case of cancer cured by exercise: Fifteen years ago, I read a cancer-cured news in a Chinese newspaper. The news shocked me. It opened my eyes to new ways of fighting cancer besides the standard treatments which I knew plenty.

The story happened in China. An elderly lady failed standard treatments for her terminal lung cancer. Her oncologist told her the ultimate sad news. She only had seven months to live.

She started running. Her husband ran with her. At first, it was a struggle just to walk. Because she was weakened after all the treatments. But they pushed on, increasing the distance of running a little bit at a time.

Seven years later, she was running seven miles everyday. The cancer? It could not be seen on CT. So the lung cancer was gone.

This was reported by a reputable Chinese newspaper that enjoys daily circulation in major cities all over the world. As an oncologist (cancer care physician), I could smell out this to be somewhat a real story.

I truly love exercise a lot and believe all the goodness it brings. But the simple act of running cured a terminal lung cancer that failed our treatments? That was unbelievable. But it sounded like a real case-history of a lung cancer patient. Nevertheless, I was still shocked and momentarily in a disbeliever mode. But I decided to do a little literature search about exercise and cancer control.

More evidence came: Before I knew, I found hundreds of reports about exercises stopping cancer in its track. There were tons of data in the web and hundreds of papers in the library. I was dumbfounded. Jesus Almighty! There is something as strong as what we oncologists can do. Before long, I also found tons of data on more lifestyle activities that can beat cancer. I was excited. These could be considered as additional treatments to the standard treatments also. Might be my patients could get better results doing these and the real treatments!

Equally strong ways to control cancer: What are these lifestyle intervention-Rx's? You know now. These are just the activities with their shocking "treatment" statistics listed in the Preface section in this book. The Preface is on the page right beneath the cover of this book. They were stress reduction, exercise, weight control and checking your vitamin D levels etc. Yahoo! I hit gold.

So I summarized those lifestyle treatments, and gave it to each patient on the consultation visit. As they say," The rest is history."

Well, in fact, those are the things I repeatedly boasted about in this book. They are not history. They can't be history. They are here to save lives!

All my patients were happy to take up those lifestyle "treatments". The summary page made them believers. A few years later. Miraculous results in my patients made me a true believer in those methods, or should I say," lifestyle intervention-Rx's" made me cry.

Patients with good cancers seemed never to recur.

So called terminal cancer patients continued to roam the earth and appeared in their primary-care doctors' offices for follow-up visits. Till their primary-care doctors noticed something odd was happening. It made them wondered, **"Boy, they shouldn't be around anymore, shouldn't they?"** the primary-care doctors mumbled to themselves, I imagined. The patients surely did exist. They were not ghosts. And they were in no hurry to go. They liked to stay around on earth for 3, 5, and 7 more years or beyond if possible.

Honestly, I myself was shocked also. How could that be?

My own patients' case histories were not as unbelievable as the case of the old lady running her lung cancer away. But they are nevertheless very encouraging. I wish to keep this book thin and inexpensive. So once again I have to refer the readers to read my other two books (*"Who isn't afraid of Cancer"; "Run...Run away from Cancer"*. If you want to read those full case histories. Type my name in the web-site Amazon.com. You will find them. And in this book, I can still briefly present relevant case-histories too. Here they are:

Case histories

Case #1: A carcinoid cancer disappeared from the lung of a patient who believed: What the patient did was just everything mentioned in this book. No medication was effective against her carcinoid cancer at the time. The mass was in the middle left lower lung field. It looked obvious and solid on chest X-ray and CT.

She received the summary paper about lifestyle "treatments" in her consultation visit. She actively lost 3 pounds in her second visit 3 months later. A couple more follow-ups later, she then was just followed up by her primary-care doctor. She had no need to be followed by me anymore. If necessary, she could be referred back to see me. And I would see her in no time.

Two years later, she somehow scheduled herself to see me again. This time, she was trying to come back just to show me the carcinoid cancer disappeared from her lung. That was obvious by pushing the button and looking at the new CT in the computer.

Silly me, I was behind schedule, was in a hurry, no time to see the glory. So I just commented," Good, it disappeared from the lung", and bid her fair-well.

Only much later, I realized she was being nice to come back and show me the little miracle. Thanks very much indeed.

Case #2: A terminal cancer patient lasting five years and more: Any cancer doctor could tell you the life-expectancy of this patient was one year. She was diagnosed with lung cancer which already had spread to the bones. I told her the same in the first visit, and gave her the paper summarizing the lifestyle "treatments". She believed in it. She bravely took the first round of chemotherapy in an attempt to control her cancer.

In her first visit, she had to come by wheelchair for the pain in the bones. The pain made it impossible to walk. She was brave, and was determined to make the best of the situation. She did as much of the lifestyle treatments as she could.

By the second visit, her pain was gone. And the wheelchair was no longer needed. Only then I realized what chemotherapy alone could not have done. But now it had been done with the help of lifestyle interventions. The fact that she could walk again without pain could not be achieved by chemotherapy alone in such a short time. She had lung cancer involving the bones. But now it was achieved. Patient was happy. I was shocked again.

She kept her weight down. She was doing exercise with her hands while sitting on her wheelchair. She lifted weights. Those weights were two large plastic soda bottles filled with water! Holy water indeed. And she was aware of calorie reduction, stress reduction etc.

She did not die at the one year mark. She lived for years like a normal person. Her family was happy like her. Though she did have to take chemotherapy every 18 months or so. The treatments plus the lifestyle "intervention-Rx's" together only slowed down the cancer.

But all those lifestyle "treatments" kept her strong. Another course of chemotherapy was effective to cut the cancer down to size and get rid of the pain, when that became necessary. She had three courses of chemotherapy in the span of five years before I retired. Treatments of chemotherapy would not have worked that well if not for her strong physical body, rejuvenated by the lifestyle intervention-Rx's. Thanks are to the lifestyle interventions.

So you know, she turned a one year survival into more than five years. I was convinced that it was lifestyle "treatments" amplifying the chemotherapy effects.

Case #3: Good-cancer patients did not seem to recur: Of the more than one thousand patients under my care annually, majority were patients with so called good cancers. They just came for routine follow-ups. I really failed to remember any cancers coming back for them. **Really, no patients of mine had cancer recurrences?**

As I was writing this statement, I tried to recall hard to the best of my efforts. I still failed to remember recurrences. It is so unbelievable that it starts to give me a dream-like feeling now. May be it really is a dream? Maybe I was getting old before retirement at that time?

Are these lifestyle habits of exercise, calorie reduction and keeping the weight down and the like, are really so potent as to make the stronger body <u>cancer-proof</u>? Or was it the time I spent there being too short to see recurrences? Only the future will tell.

Case #4: A good cancer patient stopped needing periodic treatment for years:

This patient was a late middle age lady with a good leukemia. It was called chronic lymphocytic leukemia (CLL). People live long with this leukemia, at least 95% of them. But they invariably have to be on treatments every few months; else the white blood cell number would rise right through the ceiling. (When that happened, the laboratory tech would call the on-call oncologist-hematologist with frightened voices, usually in the weird hours of midnight to 7AM. They did not know the case was not dangerous. Yes, I had a few of those.)

This patient was a little overweight. But she could not really lose any weight, hard as she tried. Yet she kept her weight constant while doing moderate exercise, stop eating when feeling 70-80% full, and she relaxed her mind very well. A year after the lifestyle "treatments" commenced. **She came off treatment for a break**. We expect the white blood cell number to go up in a few months. And to re-start treatments. <u>We waited, we waited, and we waited. The white blood cell number never went up</u>, not for the three years before I retired.

Mind you. Her CLL had a chromosome #17 mutation too. That made her CLL "Armed and dangerous". But no matter, the disease refused to get worse on her. I became a firm believer in the lifestyle interventions. For I had never seen a CLL behaved like this. I had seen more than my share of patients with CLL's dying from it after years on treatments. When the treatment no longer worked.

Case #5: A "dead men walking" family turned cheerleaders:
This case will forever remain in my fondest memories. The
patient and family -- all four of them were grown-ups. On the
first visit, they were all like "dead men walking". But for the
rest of the visits in five years, they seemed to cheer my
presence each time I saw them, minus dancing and trumpets
and drums, of course.

The patient was an elderly lady in her late 60's. She had her
colon cancer surgically removed two and a half years before. It
came back to her abdomen. It was the size of a big grapefruit.
Feeling the prominent mass, the primary doctor told her she
might only have three months to live. That news turned them
all into "dead men walking".

When I went into the room for consultation. I could not see
the patient's face. It was facing the floor, sitting in a chair,
obviously sobbing. The patient's husband and the two grown
sons were doing the same too. My heart sank.

But I assured them it might not be that bad. Because
modern treatments of chemotherapy for colon cancer had
been very effective. I handed them the paper summarizing the
lifestyle "treatments" in that first visit, not expecting much. In
fact, I joined them in the depressed world right there, just
short of crying.

We started with a mild chemotherapy pill.

Three weeks went by. I walked into the examination room
for their first follow-up visit.
I opened the door. I heard cheers! Their heads raised high.
Their faces were showing big smiles. Their eyes sparkled like
diamonds. Blessed were those happy diamonds! I thought I
heard trumpets and drums.

It turned out in three short weeks. They could not feel the
cancer anymore.

It could not be true. But that had been the fact. I totally was unprepared for that. I know that chemotherapy pill should be effective, but not that effective. But it was truly happening. I got to believe. They continued to cheer in excited voices.

Later, I figured out the lifestyle intervention-Rx's must have multiplied the chemotherapy effect. And the grapefruit size cancer shrank to an egg. I think it is a reasonable explanation.

She exercised everyday. She was cheerful, and she was healthy and kind of slim.

She was a catholic. She was going to church almost everyday alright. She had four treatments in five years till she decided not to take treatments anymore.

Thanks to the new chemotherapies. Thanks to the lifestyle "treatments" that multiplied its effect for this patient.

There were about fifteen patients in the same bad situations like her. They all did well like her, lasting for years, except four or five. Two of the young patients with lung cancers I will always remember their ways of saying "good-bye" to me in their last visits. I dedicated the last chapter to them in the other book "*Run... Run Away from Cancer.*" in Amazon.com in my name. But they were the bad exceptions. That we should not forget.

The last thing I want to add in her case. She came when she was in her 60's, and died in her early 70's, not three months as the primary doctor thought. Honestly, at first, I thought the same. I thought it was a close estimation. Never would I have expected that miracle.

Scientific Facts - At the end of reading all these facts about exercise, see if you would agree that exercise is a giant. And cancer is a dwarf?

A lot of the facts are from major studies. Though they may just appear as inconspicuously as plain simple statements. Remember it costs more than $100 millions each study producing hundreds of statements. I will put a star* on them if I remembered the studies correctly. There were hundreds of thousands of people participating in those studies also.

* *Thirty minutes of walking daily, prevents 30-40% colon cancers. It has also been proven that it prevents colon cancer and other cancers from recurrences (cancers coming back) too. *Same success-rate for prevention of recurrences for lung, breast, endometrial cancers as above. Not so for prostate cancer, it seems to need vigorous exercise. Vigorous exercise needs doctor's or expert's evaluation, but not walking.
* In another study*, exercise decrease prostate cancer deaths by 61%.
* *Three hours of walking per week, which is moderate exercise, decreases the risk of death by 34% to 67% in breast cancer studies.
*Even one hour of walking per week was found to decrease the risk of death by 40%.
* *Study showed it is Ok to start exercise after the diagnosis of cancer. On the other hand, if an active person stops exercise after cancer diagnosis, the risk would be like people who do not exercise. That means you may not get the huge benefits like those who start exercises.
* For breast cancer patients not exercising, there is a danger. Gaining weight would result in more fat cells in the body. The fat cells secrete hormones, making treatments less effective.
* Home-based exercise is Ok, like walking in the house, riding a stationary bike in front of the TV, same-place jogging over a thick cushioned mat, jumping ropes etc.

* **The more the exercise, the better the survival and the chance of cancer coming back are less. (Same conclusions from several $100-million studies.)

* Exercise releases happy hormones called endorphins. It only makes us feel happy? No, it also fights cancer in a lot of ways. The main one being that it neutralizes the stress hormones that cause cancer to spread. No spreading of the cancer, there may not be cancer deaths.

* Something you can see, though it is only in mice. When they exercise, the cancer that you can see and measure on the skin. Those cancers do not grow when the mice seemed happily running inside those drums. They ran hard, grinning as if trying to get rid of the cancer.

* Exercise increases muscle bulk. Muscle burns a lot of energy even during maintenance. We need 30 Cal a day for each gram of muscle maintenance.

* Optimal amount of exercise make the immune system stronger. The natural killer cells (NK cells) enjoy killing cancer cells more. The macrophages eat up more cancer cells for their dinners.

* Exercise is the most robust (huge) and long lasting anti-depressant known to psychological science. (Exercise is the best anti-depressant in psychological studies, and well-known to them. And the effect is long lasting.)

The danger of over-exercise: Animal studies showed over-exercise make the animal susceptible to fatal infections. In those animal experiments, The scientists gave potential fatal infections to those mice by injections. The exhausted group died a lot more than the non-exhausted group. The injected bacteria are rather "fatal" to those mice.

In humans the immune system would be weakened for 4 to 6 hours after strenuous exercise that is "over-exercise" for us. Then after 6 hours, the immune system recovers. So before the total recovery, please stay away from the crowd. Some of those people could spread an infection that can potentially be dangerous, or rarely, be fatal to you.

So after over-exercise, would it be good to stay home for 4 to 6 hours, rest or sleep, wait for your immune system to recover?

The optimal amount of exercise: It is equivalent to a total of three hours of brisk walking per week. Strictly speaking, for that, it is 9 MET-hr. But generally it is recommended to do 10 to 18 MET-hrs as optimum for the sake of exercise.

MET is metabolic equivalent task. It is the amount of energy spent or calories burned, usually measure in an hour. The following is a MET-hr table for some exercise.

1. Sitting ....1 MET-hr.
2. Slow walking ....2.3 MET-hr
3. Fast walking ....3.0 MET-hr
4. Sex ....5.8 MET-hr
5. Jogging ....7 MET-hr
6. Running ....8 MET-hr
7. Lap swimming ....8 MET-hr
8. Bicycling at moderate speed ....8 MET-hr
9. Rope jumping ....10 MET-hr

Why is exercise so powerful: There are a few dozen explanations. But I humbly would venture to vote for 3. The last one may be a new explanation from me.

1. Exercise used up the energy. So there is not enough of it left for the cancer cells. Remember the cancer cells needs 38 times the energy just for maintenance. When they do

not have enough energy, they may go into the "recycle" mode, which is known as apoptosis. As you know, when things get recycled, they don't exist any more as before.

2. Optimal amount of exercise make the immune system stronger. The natural killer cells (NK cells) enjoy killing cancer cells more. The macrophages enjoy eating up more cancer cells for lunch.

3. This last one I vote for is perhaps the best mechanical explanation. Mechanical explanation frequently is most likely to be the real explanation. On the molecular biology level - a single life is one big mechanical universe.

When we exercise, our heart rate goes up, the blood circulation speeds up. Is this mechanical enough now? Yes, it is. Wait until the time comes when the blood flow is so rapid that it flows at the "white-water-rafting" speed. What happens then?

Just think if the original cancer mass shed off cells to establish homes in another location in your body. That is scary, right. But they first have to attach to the new site. So they can undergo changes to fit in.

One scientist found out. To be successful to fit in. They need a big twelve changes. (I always wonder how they found out such things). Anyway, twelve changes may take days or months to achieve. Before that happens, they get carried away by the exercising white water speed of the blood flow. They don't have a chance to establish new home in a new location.

In fact, they most likely will meet the rapidly patrolling NK cells and macrophages, and meet their demise - killed by the NK cells or become food for the macrophages. NK cells and macrophages are immune cops patrolling the streets (blood vessels). This is way too much of a mechanical description. But that is what a real biological life is in the molecular biology world. A single life is a big mechanical universe in itself in molecular biology.

Chapter 4
Calorie Restriction (CR) - What is it? (You will learn from this chapter. It is life-or-death.)

Introduction: Calorie Restriction (CR) is a big academic term. It means stop eating when you feel 60 to 80%-full. This term CR is fondly used all the time now. Because it was found out to fight cancer very well. Most evidence showed that when a living animal (That includes us, of course) went on to a 60-80%-full dieting, the cancer population stopped growing.

Such great effect of calorie restriction is hard to imagine. Just think about it.....After eating a few mouthfuls less, the cancer slows down or stop growing? Unbelievable. That was my thinking.

But my MDS (myelodysplastic syndrome) patient's case assured me it is very believable. He almost died when he violated his self-conscious calorie-restriction, just for 2 weeks.

Please read on, you will see his case-history soon. I hope the case would help you give up the last few mouthfuls of food willingly. And form a habit of eating less.

It's just dieting - Calorie Restriction or CR: In this real world, dieting means to stop eating when one feels just a little full. It's easy to say but hard to do. But it is cancer we are fighting. So "Go do it."

It is hard to measure the percentage of food to cut away from our meals. But you are advised to learn it. Yes, learn to count calories, making total calorie about 1800 calories or less daily. Whether your cancer would come back or not. Or whether you live long or not may depend on calorie counting. You would have to know how much food to cut out. To make it easier. A dietician consultation may help.

It is good to learn the habits of counting calories. You will soon find out doing this you will keep your cancer at bay. And doing this, your family members will be aging much slower than other people. They would be looking younger.

In addition, if they do CR, they would have a greater chance of avoiding the same cancer you have. They have twice the chance of getting the same cancer than the general population.

How to live long to be 100 years old (Family member or you): This 80%-full dieting is an excellent tool to slow down aging. It has been known for hundreds of years. Benjamin Franklin had published this anti-aging effect in as early as the 1700's. It has been well proven too as you shall see in literature or the web.

But the 80%-full dieting had also been discovered to fight cancers well, besides anti-aging. The evidence is convincing. After reading the next few cases, I think you would agree.

The case of Calorie-restriction violation creating a life-and-death situation: In one of my patients, it was a matter of life-and death due to his forgetting calorie restriction for two short weeks while on vacation.

When the treatment suddenly failed to work after his vacation. We couldn't figure out what happened. We missed identifying "forgetting dieting" as the reason. It almost proved fatal. We missed it because nobody knew CR was that great.

Who would have realized that something seemed unimportant like omitting-dieting was the reason the disease turned bad? CR even was not something everybody believe in. And nobody in the world knew it was so utterly relevant and important. He went on feastings (not fasting) for two weeks and the disease went out of control. The disease almost killed him.

This book has to be brief to be inexpensive. So let's just briefly mention his case.(It is very detail in my other book," *Run.... Run Away from Cancer*") - Amazon.com and type in my name. In that book, look for it in the chapter on MDS.

This patient had a myelodysplastic syndrome (MDS). He had bad cells in his bone marrow, where blood cells are made. The bad cells could not mature right, though they grew just a little faster than normal. He had very low and quickly falling red blood cells, white blood cells and platelets.(Not just mildly low and stable which is not dangerous.) His blood counts could and did drop very low quickly.

In a couple of days, he became energy deficient due to low red cells not bringing enough oxygen for energy production.

More dangerous than that, his low platelets numbers made him bleed automatically. He had to rush to the emergency room when that happened. Just imagine he could bleed to death or bleed in the brain with the danger of a disabling stroke. Let's back up to the beginning.

Now you get the picture. At first, he had been getting transfusions weekly, or twice weekly. He was like living in the emergency room. That was a very miserable life.

But two molecularly designed drugs came to his rescue, saved his life and let him avoid the messy bleedings and transfusions. In fact his life was almost normal. He continued to work as a VIP in his firm.

The first drug was working well till he went to London, England. He feasted there with his friends on fine English cuisines for two weeks.

When he came back to California, He started to nose-bleed . We did not know why the drug failed. Oh, please wait a minute, the drug was supposed to fail for everyone after using it for 6 months. That was known for MDS patients under treatment with the two drugs.

But he had been doing well for almost two years. Because he had been doing the lifestyle "intervention-Rx's". That must have helped the drug to control the disease for more than 6 months. Thus the treatment effect was amplified 4 times or more already.

There were too many unknown reasons for the drug to fail right after traveling to London.

Fortunately, the second molecular drug worked. Then 18 months later, he drove to Ohio and feasted on those fresh farm foods. The second drug failed after he came back.

At that moment, we spent time during the follow-up visit to discussed what the reason was. We concluded it was most likely the feasting of food. Because there was no other reasons we could think of. He thought he ran out of treatment options, summoned his daughter from Southern California to spend his last days in San Francisco with him!

But fortunately, I dug up a reported case from the literature, the combination of the two drugs worked. Life was again back to normal. I bet from there on, it was to be no feasting in his life. He remained transfusion free for 4 years. Then I retired.

Proposed mechanism why calorie restriction worked in this case of the MDS patient (myelodysplastic syndrome patient) : Please note the mechanism is my reasoning from the scientific knowledge of basic hematology (the study of blood diseases), and from college biochemistry. (This case might be the first case treated this way and lasted so long).

I think the bad cell populations needed more energy to grow - tons of energy. When tons of energy was not available while he was strictly dieting, they didn't grow. The good cells took over, and provide sufficient good matured cells in the blood. Dieting and other lifestyle intervention-Rx's might have made the molecular drugs keep on working, way over its effective time limit of half a year. Six months was the time the drug supposed to fail. So the fact that the blood count had been normalized for years was impossible for the drug alone. The drug was still working for 2 years at one point, and 18+ months at another, was mainly because of the lifestyle intervention-Rx's helped the drug effectively.

But feasting supplied enough energy for the bad cell populations to grow a little faster, and outnumbered the normal cells, and making the molecular drug useless. The result was the bad cells took over. They didn't mature well and the blood count dropped like a stone. The platelets number became so low that the patient bled and almost died.

Case-histories: Calorie-restriction controlling cancer was known for more than a 100 years too. We have seen the power of this simple 80%-dieting in the case we just discussed now let's see more: (The Nobel Prize case showed the mechanism why CR works).

Historic Nobel Prize event: Otto Warburg, a physiologist and physician, found out cancer cells were clumsy. They made energy inefficiently - He received a Nobel Prize in 1931 for that. He found the predominant glycolysis environment in cancer cells. Glycolysis is one way to make energy (ATP) from sugar (glucose). In this glycolytic pathway, 1 glucose makes 1 ATP (One sugar makes one energy unit). This is important for understanding CR.

Evolution had fitted out our cells with a more modern way of making energy - the tricarboxylic acid cycle where one sugar produces 38 energy units. This is a 38 times the difference in energy production.

Cancer cells degenerates. It loses the modern way of making energy and only has the glycolytic pathway left - one sugar, one energy unit. So they need 38 times the amount of sugar to produce the same amount of energy a cell needs, do they? I put the question mark there as to show this is from my own reasoning. Not a theory from the books.

Though, it is a matter of fact that cancer cells do need lots of sugar. And it's just as easy not to give them enough sugar, so they may die. I will show later in the last paragraph of this chapter that cancer cells do take a lot of sugar.

But it is utterly true, no energy, no cancer growth. We will see that in the cases below.

Case #1: No food, no cancer growth: More than 150 years ago, it was observed in mice with cancer growing on the skin. Giving the mice less food, the cancer in the mice stopped growing. Less food can make the cancer stop growing. Is calorie-reduction simple and wonderful? So it helps to remember," No food, no cancer growth." while you go on dieting merrily. Isn't it worthwhile, be mildly hungry in brief moments of the day, but may put the cancer away?

What are those extra food? Those food that we can put away to make the 80% full dieting? Those food are in our last few mouthfuls when eating. Sacrifice them. Let the cancer cells go hungry too but they may die. This is the beauty of calorie restriction.

As for us humans, when feeling a little hungry, drink several spoonfuls of soup, or a few sips of milk or soy-milk, or even plain water. A few roasted nuts may help too. Our hungry feeling would be suppressed till the regular 80% full diet is ready later.

Case #2: 80% full dieting, live to be a 100 year old: It was a year in the 1970's. A respected science journal published a finding. <u>In an island, people lived more than 100 years old easily</u>.

That was in the 1970's. The average age was 65 years old or so.

All the interested scientists flocked to the island. (I wanted to go too. But I wasn't even in college). Well, they did their research, came up with lots of explanations. (Boy, arguments!)

But the final solid reason was finally agreed upon. People who live in that island have the firm custom of "eating till 80% full".

There were 740 people older than 100 years old in a population of 1.3 million people. That island is Okinawa Island in Japan. They have detailed population records in Japan. This was in the official record. That was extreme longevity at the time (Ain't no aliens). But did they have less cancers too?

Yes they did have much less cancers:

~ Breast cancers were 50% less than other place.
~ Prostate cancers were 50% less than us.
~ Colon cancers were even less than 50% compared to us.
~ Ovarian cancers were less than 50% as well.

Case #3: A historical case of eating less, getting less cancers in USA: That happened in the 1930's. It was the worst of times. But it was the best of times for cancer statistics.

That was the time of the "great depression". Food was scarce. People ate sparingly. And they had less cancers. The number of cancers was 120 compared to 174 per 100k people in other better times.

In the good times nowadays, the number of cancer has been increasing. It won't take long before it doubles in number. Plenty of food and obesity is going to kill more of us.

Case #4: Monkeys given 80% food only, has 50% less cancers: That is surprising. How could this happen? This probably is due to the fact that there was not extra-energy (sugar) that the cancer cells needed for survival and growth. So 50% of the monkeys' cancers never had a chance to grow and show.

Case # 5: Less food in humans, 50% less cancers: This case was reported by a surgeon who did stomach bypass surgeries. Food eaten through the mouth, by-passed the stomachs, making those people absorb very little food. They kept themselves thin. There were 84 of his patients like that. What was the cancer rate ten years down the line?

The surgeon reported they had 50% less cancers than the general population. The same 50% reduction in cancers just like the monkeys on diet.

So the scientists are right. We must be related, monkeys and us humans.

Case #6: **Benjamin Franklin -** In 1733, Benjamin Franklin wrote in his then very popular publication "Poor Richard's Almanac" the following," To lengthen thy (your) life, lessen thy meals." His pen-name was Poor Richard.

Poor Richard? Poor master Franklin! There were no high-paying speech-circuits at that time. He would have been very rich if he lives in to-day's world, like those big-shot politicians now, giving speeches for $$$$$ every week or so.....

And should he have known that dieting had been proven anti-cancers too. He might write elaborately, extensively, and incessantly on the topic and would have made himself one of the greatest authors in American history.

Well, he already had left his indelible name in American history. And <u>you can't easily find a man more lightning-proof than him</u>.

Oh yes, my patients' cases: One case we have already discussed. That was the MDS (myelodysplastic syndrome) man who almost died when he released his calorie-restriction. That one case is enough to show us how serious it is to stop eating when we just feel a little full. It showed also amply how powerful lifestyle interventions-Rx's are.

I know the feeling when I eat about 70% of the amount of food I used to eat. My wife had some dietician training as an RN. Anyway, that was all she cooked for me and no more. I got used to that portion and know it when feeling a little full. It's 70% and no more.

But for you, counting calorie till you know when to stop at 70-80% full is going to be a learning process. It may take sometime. But you'll be there. Please start with calories counting. Eventually, it may be life-saving . i.e. Your dear life.

The other case is also a patient with myelodysplastic syndrome (MDS). Her case was much less dramatic. She had a busy job. Human interactions were a major part of her work. She was also a VIP. She had to look good. So she strictly obeyed dieting.

Her MDS (myelodysplastic syndrome) never went out of control. She should have failed the two drugs and died of infection or bleeding in a year or so. This was the "natural" course for MDS patients in her serious stage treated with the two drugs that would lose effectiveness over time. Or the disease would grow resistant to it over time.

But her life remained normal. The first molecular drug at 80% dose was keeping her life normal for 5 years before I retired. Her lucky survival was mainly due to her dieting.

As you know now, dieting makes the difference between life-or-death. And dieting is an important part of the "treatments" for this particular stage of the MDS patients. <u>I just wish all the MDS patients in their same "stages" know about these stories and give dieting a serious try</u>.

Convincing facts: They are mostly scientific, mostly from human calorie-restriction studies.

* In mice, there is a model of human breast caner. 70% full dieting, the number of metastasis (spreading) to the lungs was much lower.
* 80% full dieting reduced the amount of the hormones and anabolic steroids, slowing down the rate of cancer growth.
* 80% full dieting reduced the level of natural chemicals for cell-growth.
* 80% full dieting reduced the inflammation stateinour body. The inflammatory state is a warm-bed for cancer growths.
* 80% full dieting reduced oxidative stress that could cause cancer.
* 80% full dieting decreased the rate of cell division. Uncontrolled cell division is the hallmark of cancer.
* 80% dieting boosted the immune cells that are supposed to go eating or killing cancer cells.
* 80% full dieting increased our power to repair damaged cells. Millions of millions of cells are damaged in our body daily. Damaged cells could give rise to cancer.
* In mice, 30% less food plus treatments reduced the number of cancer metastasis (spreading). And the size of the metastasis was smaller.
* 80% dieting causes our body to switch off some genes while activating others. This, as researchers found, switched our body from growth phase to maintenance phase. Gene modes switching sounds logical. On maintenance mode, growth probably is halted or slowed down.

Why does calorie-restriction (80% full dieting) work? All the findings in the Convincing Facts section probably all help to stall cancer.

But I think the major difference is the 38 times less energy generated out of one unit of sugar (glucose). For this inefficiency in generating energy, the cancer cell needs lots of glucose. They accumulate so much glucose. When the glucose was made radioactive before giving it to the patients. The cancers absorb most of the radioactive glucose. They will light up for the PET scan. This is basic science.

If you do not give cancer cells enough energy. They may die. The scientists have shown when they lack energy to grow, the cancer cells know it's time to go away. Cells including cancer cells, go away by a recycle-program called apoptosis, or programmed cell death. The unwanted cells or the old cells break down the large molecules inside the cell, and wrap the pieces up in small vesicles and disappears. Those vesicles are picked up by growing cells. Your cancer cells die!

So do not give them energy (sugar). Just eat till you are 60-80% full. You then have barely enough to live (Yes, poor me. But got to do it.). And the energy available may not have 38 times the energy for the cancer cells. They may die. That is what you want, right?

Chapter 5
Weight control - It is worth the Sacrifice

Introduction: Why is weight-control worth the sacrifice?
Because it is proven to control cancer.

Let's ask ourselves a question. There are more and more people getting over-weight. And there are more and more people come down with cancers. Can there be a connection?

I am afraid the answer is Yes. <u>Obese people have more cancers</u>. This has been recognized for a while - a few decades perhaps.

Obesity is common all over the world now. Two third of the people in the US are obese. So is the rest of the world perhaps. So the number of cancers is increasing in the world. This means more and more people are having increasing fat cells in the bodies. What can fat do to us? Let's look at some case-histories.

Case-histories:

Case #1: My young obese patient went down early: This was a sad case. He was a lively young man. He was not obese at the beginning of the chemotherapy-course that took a year in the old days. Now it is only a few months of treatments for stage 3 colon cancer.

He had a 60% chance of cure. Even if he was not cured. The cancer could be controlled for a few years. He should have 2-3 years of life if the cancer was not cured.

He kept on gaining weight over the year despite me begging him each time he came for chemotherapy. It was to no avail sadly. By the end of the treatments, he became a "butter-ball" as they called it.

He died 3 months after treatment completion.

In gaining weight and becoming very obese, he gave up the 60% chance of cure. If not cured. There was to be several years to live. He gave that up too.

Now as I am writing up his case. I still feel like it is the end of the world, how depressing.

This happened in New York, before I handed out the lifestyle intervention-Rx's papers to patients in California, about 20 years later.

The time was in the early 1990's. Those research reports of reducing stress, calorie reduction, weight control and exercise, all could fight cancer, had not been commonly published in cancer journals yet.

Case #2:Losing 3 pounds, the carcinoid cancer disappeared: This is a case I love to repeat telling.

The case was a middle age lady who was a little bit overweight. She had a ping-pong size mass at the left lower lung. There was no effective treatment for carcinoid tumor at that time. She took up the lifestyle interventions/treatments of weight control etc. She did lose 3 pound in the follow-up visit. Two years later. The mass was not there anymore by CT.

Case #3: A fearful breast cancer lost its grip of death: Lose 5 pounds and maintained it for 10 years, there were 50% more survivors. This was from a world famous study. The results were squeezed out from a sub-group analysis, reported in 2015 in the news.

This is 50% more survivors from one of the worst kind of breast cancers. It is called "Triple negative" breast cancer. So called because it is negative for some molecular structures called the estrogen receptor, the progesterone receptor and the Her2 receptor.

The name "Triple negative" does indeed sound like something evil. But it still does not convene its awfulness and ugliness. And if you know normally 90% of the regular breast cancer patients are cured. And in these triple-negative breast cancer patients, there is only a 50% chance of cure. You know it is a cancer with a firm death-grip on half the people.

Terrible cancer, half the people die. So out of 100 ladies with tripe-negative breast cancers, 50 of them would die. But actively losing 5 pounds, 25 more of those young ladies would become alive. I am sure they did other lifestyle interventions like exercise, calorie reduction etc to be able to keep the weight down.

It is not easy to keep the weight down. But doing that to beat cancers is well worth the while. You get your life back, and win the battle against cancer.

Winning the battle against cancer is always some thoughts to cherish, to enjoy for the rest of your life.

Come on, let's do these things: Since the whole world is recommending weight control! Let's make it easy for us to do. So we can face the organizations that recommend this thing called weight control. These organizations, they are the heart, cancer, government, and the world health organizations etc. So let's just spring into actions, and form a habit of those actions and try these actions. We want to be good citizens of the world:

1. Get up and walk whenever we can. I think that is the easiest of the exercises. It's fun to walk on the street, and say "Hello" in your heart to the trees and birds. In the botanical gardens, you can walk and learn the names of trees, shrubs, or flowers. You can walk on the beaches and say hello to the sea gulls. But there are places not safe to walk.

Californians, please don't go walking outside the city too far, and ending up saying hello to mountain lions. They may be hungry. I have many lion stories, but not going to talk about them here. Please go jog somewhere else. We can keep our weight down safely too.

2. Another easy and fun exercise. It is to ride the stationary bike in front of the T.V. We can finish one movie and burn 300 calories in one sitting. A few of those per week. We could lose a few pounds.

3. You have mild back pain? I do. To get rid of it. I just plant my feet on the floor at home, standing, and swing my arms and turn my body gently from side to side. If I count 300 times, it may just be 5 minutes. By then, my back pain would be gone.

Remember? If we do one hour of this in a week while watching TV, instead of sitting on the sofa. We may achieve a 40% reduction in the chance of death from cancer. Even though that statistics was supposed to be walking, not swinging arms around the body.

4. Please do no snack: This is the number one reason we gain weight. It's from studies.

5. What happen when we are hungry between meals? Drink milk or soy milk. They fill up the stomach and erase the hungry feeling for a while. Water can do it too, but it won't last .

6. Eat plenty of vegetables. Their fibers fill the stomach up but bring only a few calories.

7. Eating is a pleasure. But if we eat till we feel full and rub our bellies. That is too much food. You may gain weight. Studies show that after we eat. It takes 20 minutes to feel full. So get a habit of not eating till you feel full.

8. If we don't eat till we feel full, we may look very young even after we retired. That sounds like a good deal to make. You have decades of golden "young" "slim" days ahead of you.

These are the few things that come to my mind. Form a habit and you may keep your weight down and beat cancer. Let's get some encouragement from the facts section now. It may make losing a few pounds easier.

Convincing facts: Weight lost, cancer lost:

*American Cancer Society says: If you lose weight, or keep from gaining weight, plus exercise and good food diet. You survive longer and you decrease your chance of cancer coming back (Recurrence).
*The American Cancer Society has guidelines for exercise and nutrition in the website:www.cancer.org/NUPA.
*Increased weight leads to increased fat cells which make more estrogens. People would have more cancers of the breast, colon, prostate, and endometrium and more.
*Overweight leads to more glucose (sugar) in blood. Cancer cells have more fuel to grow.
*Overweight leads to increased inflammatory state in the body, setting up a warm bed for cancers to start and grow.
*Observational studies report recently: (Observing humans)
        .Active weight loss results in less cancer recurrence by 30-40%.

One thing that helped me keeps the weight down:
To state it simply, is to bear with mild feeling of hunger willfully. But it is very hard to bear with the feeling and not to find food. I usually go drink water or soy milk. Since I have lactose intolerance. I also take some nuts. These food controls hunger longer.

Chapter 6
Sugar feeds Cancers

Introduction: "Sugar feeds cancers" is accepted by Europeans. In USA, some people are skeptical about it.

There are a few dozens reasons why sugar feeds cancers. But two basic facts make me a firm believer.

1. Sugar is acidic. In this acidic environment in our body when sugar in our blood is aplenty. Those brave cells that fight cancers do not work well. Like macrophages are cells that eat cancer cells for lunch. If the blood is high in sugar, they work 50% of their might. May be, 50% of cancer cells could escape in this situation. But at the least, high sugar in blood would let cancer establish itself easier since now they then can get enough sugar.

2. Cancer cells end people's lives when they spread to critical organs. They spread through highway 12-LOX in mice breast cancer cell models, with the sugar levels in the Western diets. That highway lets cancer cells spread to the lungs.

Though this is only a study with mice model of human breast cancers. There is the similar highway in humans too when sugar is high. You'll see the fact soon.

Case-histories of real persons are always more convincing. Here it comes.

Case-histories: Case #1: A fat young man died before his time: He was an average-weight young man at the beginning of the year long treatment. He had stage 3 colon cancer. The treatment in the early 1990's when he was being treated was 12 long months, one day per month (I think I remember correctly). He kept on gaining weight, seen eating a lot of candies while waiting for his chemotherapy. He must have been doing that at home too.

I advised him not to gain weight. Gaining weight and getting more cancer was well-known at that time. But not too many studies proved gaining weight are bad for people with cancer. But I knew It was bad. So I advised him to keep his weight down. He kept on gaining weight.

Later, I became begging him not to gain weight as he was slowly looking like a bear. By the end of the 12 months, he was round. People called him "butterball". That shape was sad to look at. But little did I know how bad it influenced his survival. Death was knocking outside his door.

A short 3 months after treatment. I heard he passed away. Then I knew it was extremely bad to gain a lot of weight with cancer. And now I know the candies he ate supplied all the energy the cancer needed to grow and brushed away the might of chemotherapy. And it took his life away. Now plenty of studies proved those two points - sugar feeds cancer, and gaining weight means earlier death with cancer.

Why should I say he died before his time. He certainly did. If he was cured, which he had a 60% chance in those days. He would live a few decades more. Should he failed the treatment, he still should live another 2 or 3 years before the end.

But he died in just 3 short months. He gave up all his time in exchange for the candies he ate.

Skeptics. Did sugar feed cancer?

Case #2. A very sad case: Nowadays with liver cancer, CT picks them up early. People with liver cancers either can be cured or they can live many a years even when not cured. The molecular drugs once again came to the need for life-prolongation for patients with liver cancer. (There is less side-effects with them too). This case happened long before the molecular drugs came on the scene.

This is a case of a young lady diagnosed with unresectable (not able for surgical cutting and curing) liver cancer. Some patients died within weeks if the cancer was very aggressive.

This young lady's liver cancer was aggressive. I could feel several egg-size masses over the liver. They were rock-hard.

There was a strong combination chemotherapy. We did the treatment as inpatient for her because that old chemotherapy was too strong for patients to take coming from home. Even though it was in a small city 40 minutes outside San Francisco. And usually there was no traffic jams. Life was easier there.

Five days of chemotherapy turned the cancer masses small and soft. She had to take 3 days to recover in the hospital. Relatives and fiends were coming from all over the world to spend time with her. She was a local celebrity.

She was skin-and-bones. We both agreed. With that appearance, when dozens of people coming to see her at home was not nice. So we agreed on a little fluid hydration and nutrition. The nutrition fluid contained quite a bit of sugar and carbohydrate that could quickly turn into sugar (glucose). Those stuff could feed cancer, we only knew vaguely about it at that time.

The next morning when I was doing my morning round, the cancer masses were big and rock-hard again, though not as big as they were before treatment. She could feel them herself then. The IV fluid was stopped and the lines were out on her request even before I arrived in her room. She sat there, sad, dejected, and broken hearted.

Who wouldn't be broken hearted? She went through hell to complete the chemotherapy. The rock hard cancer softened after a week's treatment. But one night with the nutrition fluid that contained a lot of sugar, the softened liver cancer masses turned rock hard again. This nutrition fluid with sugar was like poison from Satan. It fed the devilish cancer. Sugar started to frighten me very much since that case. It was burned into my memory.

She did look a little less skinny and dry. But both she and I were feeling awful. How could soft smaller masses grew overnight to be bigger and rock-hard? Did the sugar feed the cancer! Did the nutrition fluid feed the cancer! We wished we knew beforehand. But........But it was too late! If the fluid continued, she would be dead in a few days.

She went home. Definitely by then she knew to continue dieting, though she was very thin. She took in just enough calories and nutrition. So she did not die in one week.

Four months later, She passed away. The newspaper published the news of her passing. It took a full page of the local newspaper. An accomplished and shinning life had vanished just like that. Cancer took another life this time, a brilliant life, just like that.

I almost cried when I saw that page of newspaper. I never even could calm myself down to read the paper. I never read it.

Please, please don't tell me sugar does not feed cancer! Please don't make me cry.

Convincing facts:

* Cancer cells need a lot of sugar. Give them less, they may die by recycling (Apoptosis). Do we want to withhold sugar to kill cancer cells? Yes, give them no sugar if possible. The transformed cancer cells degenerate usually and lose the modern energy production mechanism (Tricarboxylic acid cycle) and use only the ancient mechanism (glycolysis). The ancient mechanism produces only one energy from one unit of sugar. But normal cells with both mechanisms make 38 units of energy from one sugar.

The cancer cells need a lot of sugar. Not giving it to them may stall their growth, or induce them to die by recycling (Apoptosis). Normal cells would be Ok.

* Diabetic patients have higher sugar levels in the blood. They have more cancers of each type. They have more deaths from the same type of cancers.

*There was a study of more than 100,000 people without diabetics but their sugar levels were higher. The ones with higher sugar levels developed more cancers.

* Higher sugar levels in the blood would trigger inflammatory state. That is a warm-bed for cancer development and growth. Remember, obesity brings this state too.

* More than 1000 people with colon cancers were studied. The ones with higher sugar levels have more cancers coming back. And more of them died of the cancers often.

* In an animal model of breast cancer, sugar built the cancer spreading pathway for cancer to go to the lungs, the 12-LOX pathway.

* In human prostate cancer cells, if you shut off the 12-LOX pathway, the cancer cells went into the re-cycle mode (apoptosis, or programmed cell death) and disappeared. Human interventional studies may be on the way.

* In one fasting studies (taking food every other day only), the people with cancer in this study only ate every other day. (I am sure the calories and the sugar they took in is much less than normal). The result showed the cancer growth was much less. And less of these people died of cancer. (Apparently nobody died of hunger). There have been a few of those studies.

Obvious conclusion: So if you don't give enough sugar to the cancer cells. Your cancer may not grow or come back, and they could even die by re-cycling (Apoptosis).

Chapter 7
Vitamin D and Cancer Prevention

Introduction:Why just talk about vitamin D. While there are so many supplements. This is a good question. It deserves a good answer.

It's because it has been well-proven low vitamin D level in the blood is associated with a chance of getting cancer. All the other supplements may be good and necessary, and anti-cancer. But unfortunately, some supplements have been proven in international human trials to cause cancer. So the researchers were "burned" and shocked.

So the recommendation officially, world-wide: NO SUPPLEMENTS.

Vitamin D is recommended if the level in the blood is low.

Why discuss vitamin D: Because studies convinced almost everybody that it can prevent cancer. It can prevent cancer in individuals who have low vitamin D levels in the blood. If they take vitamin D supplement, they probably will prevent some cancers.

So when the vitamin D level in the blood is low in you. It should be better to take vitamin D to prevent cancer. But it is necessary to start it with your doctor so he can check the blood level of vitamin D later.

Who has low vitamin D? Me or may be you too. Low vitamin D level in blood has been found in 75% of the people in one study. So testing for vitamin D level is a very sound advice and perhaps a necessary test. It is estimated that 50,000 to 70,00 people die from cancers yearly because of low vitamin D levels.

How was vitamin D found to prevent cancer? How did this come by? I just pulled data from memory of the oncology studies I did a few decades ago. It might be a little bit off, especially in this old brain. But it will make the readers understand vitamin D. For that we have to go back a few decades in the old days.

In the old days, people in the North (like Yankees) were found to have more lymphomas - cancers of the lymphatic system. Lymphomas used to be deadly in the past, no more now.

Then the reason why Yankees had more lymphomas was found to be related to low vitamin D level. Further studies revealed that for people in the South, they have more sun-exposure and higher vitamin D level in the blood.

Sunshine on our skin makes us feel happy. John Denver even sang songs about that. It also produces vitamin D, after the uv-B of the sunshine shines on our skin. So whoever has less sunshine has less vitamin D in the blood. Those were people in the North. And they had more lymphomas than people in the South. But now vitamin D supplement may have changed the North/South difference.

Later thousands of studies all point to people with low vitamin D in blood, have more cancers. People with high vitamin D level in the blood, have less cancers of all kinds.

As an example, this finding could be seen in a report in the year 1980. People with high vitamin D level in the blood, have only 50% of the colon cancers than people with low vitamin D level.

Later on, more population studies showed that having an adequate level of vitamin D protects against other cancers like cancers of the breast, prostate, and pancreas etc.

Is high level of vitamin D necessary?

Since high levels of vitamin D seemed protective of cancers. Everybody is pushing their vitamin D level high in the blood at one point. Betting it would be proven high level of vitamin D in blood is necessary to protect against cancers. But 5 to 10 years have passed now. No proof that one needs high level of vitamin D has been published.

Yet side-effects of vitamin D taken along with calcium gave quite a few people stones in the kidney and other soft tissues. The pain of stones in the kidneys scares the vitamin takers. The pain in the kidney caused by stone is so severe. It causes people to sweat profusely, and double themselves up. Of course it is treatable in the hospital. But people starts keeping normal levels of vitamin D, waiting for decision from studies whether high level of vitamin D is necessary or not.

Bad side effects of too high a vitamin D intake along with calcium: Vitamin D makes calcium absorption into the body easier. Higher calcium level in blood can give rise to stones in soft tissues. Stone in the kidneys we've just talked about.

If stones deposit in the heart, it can cause irregular beats (rhythm). Irregular rhythms can be dangerous.

My vitamin D level was low. So I started taking vitamin D capsules daily, pushing it to higher than current upper level. But years went by, and there has been no proof that we need higher level. So now I am taking a dose to produce high normal level in blood.

Old folks have more falls when taking vitamin D: Recently, old folks taking vitamin D were found to have more falls. Some falls resulted in serious injuries.

While I was taking high dose vitamin D in the past. I sometimes find myself having problems balancing myself while walking. When it happened, I had a loss of position sense temporarily. Thank goodness for my athletic ability. It gave me quick motor reactions to re-balance myself. I never fell. That's the advantage of doing exercise routinely.

But I would agree with the above findings of taking vitamin D makes old folks fall easier.

Convincing facts:

* 75% of the people are low or deficient in vitamin D.
* In colon cancer patients, the fact is clear. At high level of vitamin D in blood, there is only half the chance of getting colon cancer.
*Vitamin D encourages the immature cells to mature up. Immature cells can turn cancerous.
* Vitamin D also prevents the immature cells from turning cancerous.
* Vitamin D stops cell from (blindly) dividing. Cancer cells divide without stop.
* Vitamin D stops new blood vessels to be formed. Cancer cells need to form new blood vessels for nutrition to divide and grow.
* Normal clothing prevents skin from making sufficient vitamin D. And too much uv-B would cause skin cancers. So supplements are the way to go if your blood level is low.
* The dose to take is less than 5000 IU's (international unit) per day, as an official recommendation. But only blood level tests after taking vitamin D for a while, is the way to decide how much to take.
* It is estimated that 50,000 to 70,000 people die from cancer yearly because of low vitamin D levels.

* More and more studies showed vitamin D is important for the immune system. The immune system is the system responsible for stopping cancers in us.

* When people are diagnosed with breast or colon cancer, they have more advanced stages if their blood vitamin D levels are low.

* 75% of patients with breast, prostate, lung, thyroid, and colon cancers have low vitamin in their blood.

*Vitamin D helps un-needed cells to recycle themselves by the program called apoptosis.

* When prostate cancer gets worse, the blood test called PSA goes up. Vitamin D slows down the rise of PSA.

Chapter 8
Supplements, Vegetable-mainly diet, Low fat diet, low cholesterol and cancer

Introduction: Let's remind ourselves with a question. What can we do to prevent lung cancers? Then I would mention a few supplements that made cancer appear/grow in human gold-standard trials.

I got the answer right. Stop smoking will prevent 80% of the lung cancers.

Vegetables-mainly diets: Yes they can prevent cancers if you eat plenty of them daily. Of course it is necessary to eat proteins, and a little fat too.

Every vegetable we eat is anti-cancer. These findings have been proven. Studies that proved them were usually couples of decades old. So the health authorities have long term data. They could see adequate proofs of the anti-cancer effect.

So there was the official recommendation more than a decade ago: Five servings of salads a day. While I read this recommendation when I was busy working. I felt only the cows can do this leisurely. They can graze all day and do nothing else.

But now I do eat mainly vegetable diets, mostly cooked. 60% of my food is vegetable. This habit cured my irritable bowels. But I am not sure this fits everybody.

Supplements that made cancer grow: I wish to write this book brief. So it could be inexpensive. For details, there is a whole chapter on supplements in one of my other 2 books: "...Run away from Cancer". This is the basis for **"no supplements".**

In those human studies, it was "pure stuff, and at high dose" pills etc. So if we eat the foods that contain them at low levels, there should be no problem of "making cancers grow". In fact, some authors even recommend, "If you really want to take supplements, take a recommended dose may be Ok."

Most of these adverse events were found accidentally and shockingly in gold-standard human clinical trials - those supplements were highly anti-cancer in laboratory studies. But showed opposite effect in large human studies. They are:
1. Beta-carotene: It grew human lung cancers in a world famous study.
2. Folate, or folic acid: It grew colon cancer in one big human study.
3. Selenium and vitamin E: Human prostate cancer grew or appeared.
4. High fish-oil level in blood was found to be associated with prostate cancer.
5. Even daily-vitamin was found to have a very small increase in cancers. But this result is very weak and not convincing.

Some supplements I have to take:
1. I take B12 daily. My blood level was low. It might have been low because I have been taking Metformin, a glucose lowering drug. It fights cancer very well too and are in several human studies now. (Please see my other book: "*Run...Run away from cancer.*)
2. I am taking Biotin daily too for my dry skin, and in the hope it can prevent my hair from thinning. It seemed to work. I am not bald yet.
3. I am taking vitamin D daily because my blood level was very low.
4. I do take daily-vitamin about 2 times a week because of my mainly vegetable diet.
5. I take calcium, low dose now and then. My blood calcium was once on the low normal side.

What does low-fat diet has to do with cancer? Indeed people on low-fat diet have less cancers. Most doctors and experts think it is not the low fat itself. Or at least not low-fat diet alone. People taking low-fat diet are usually health-conscious. They exercise, they stop eating when feeling a little full, or even before feeling full. Of course, they try to keep their weight down and check their vitamin D levels.

Now you have no doubt all these things they do are powerful lifestyle intervention-Rx's against cancer. No wonder then, people on low-fat diets have fewer cancers.

Vegetable mainly diet and low red meat diet: There is enough evidence that vegetable-mainly dieting people have lower cancer risk. The red meat diet had been linked to colon cancer.

Low cholesterol causes more cancers?

For decades, low cholesterol level was said to be possibly associated with getting more cancers. When one big report came out about 10 years ago, showing low total cholesterol is associated with more cancers. The researchers were frank and honest. They mentioned the Chinese people have low cholesterol levels, but they have fewer cancers. Meaning to me, it probably is not the cause. But some others reasons unknown, is responsible for the association. Or it may happen only in a sub-population of people.

Before that report, it has been observed for decades that low cholesterol levels in males is associated with 30% increased risk of cancers.

Recently, a report showed a more consistent association with lung and colon cancers in men. It is less clear in women whether low cholesterol level is associated with cancer or not.

A Japanese study found that medications lowering cholesterol may add to cancer risk. The lowest total cholesterol group had more cancers.

The nutritional guideline has dropped the requirement for how little cholesterol has to be present in a diet. That is good news for beacon- and egg-lovers like me.

So now "low cholesterol may be causing cancer" is in some authors' minds.

The Framingham Study (US) has been following cholesterol (and heart disease) in its study population for about half a century now. This study has revealed a lot of cardiovascular health findings. As low cholesterol is concerned, their data showed low cholesterol could predate the cancers for years. They thought low cholesterol itself does not cause cancer, but oddly it just could predate cancer (Typical academic jargons).

Each and every researcher in this group has been keen on lowering cholesterol.

Now that lowered cholesterol could predate (bring) cancer. They are really facing a big dilemma in their lives," To be or not to be. Eat the bacon or drop the bacon?" that is the question. Isn't this same question important for us all!

For me, my total cholesterol is low. So I always like the pre-cooked bacon, thick and without preservatives.

I believe the liver synthesize cholesterols for the body to use. There is a purpose for the cholesterols. We know we need them for a lot of cellular functions. And yet we have been trying to lower the total cholesterol. could this be right? May be it is just the ratio of the cholesterols went wrong to cause the cardiovascular problems?

May be we are still missing something? I am not an expert in this problem. But in blood diseases studies, it is pointed out microscopic "wounds" in the blood vessels initiate the clotting and cause ischemia. What could we do to prevent those wounds from happening?

To me, something can help people with cancers. We can at least let patients try these lifestyle interventions as part of the cancer therapy. And if found effective (in trials?), they should be incorporated into standard treatments for cancer patients.

We are talking about a very probable great recurrence reductions and great life-prolongations. Isn't that the true spirit of medicine-for-humanity?